How to Vegan

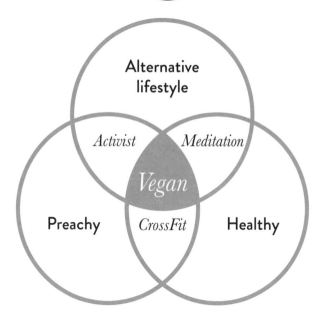

Alternative lifestyle

Activist *Meditation*

Vegan

Preachy *CrossFit* Healthy

Bitch, Peas

Stephen Wildish

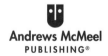

Andrews McMeel
PUBLISHING®

Andrews McMeel Publishing
a division of Andrews McMeel Universal
1130 Walnut Street, Kansas City, Missouri 64106

www.andrewsmcmeel.com

First published in 2020 by Pop Press, an imprint of Ebury Publishing,
20 Vauxhall Bridge Road,
London SW1V 2SA

20 21 22 23 24 TEN 10 9 8 7 6 5 4 3 2 1

ISBN: 978-1-5248-6082-0

Library of Congress Control Number: 2020930778

Editor: Jean Z. Lucas
Art Director: Holly Swayne
Production Manager: Carol Coe
Production Editor: David Shaw

ATTENTION: SCHOOLS AND BUSINESSES
Andrews McMeel books are available at quantity discounts with bulk purchase for
educational, business, or sales promotional use. For information, please e-mail the
Andrews McMeel Publishing Special Sales Department:
specialsales@amuniversal.com.

Have I told you I'm vegan yet?

Contents

Introduction

Answers to questions like:
"What is a vegan, wait, I don't eat
gluten, am I a vegan?!" and more.

Introduction

Welcome to *How to Vegan*, a guide to being a vegan.
Contrary to popular belief, going vegan is pretty easy. You don't need
any special equipment or a uniform. Those things are available, sure,
but they are not a requirement.

We will cover how to eat vegan, how to talk vegan, and how to cope
with people in bars who don't understand nutrition.

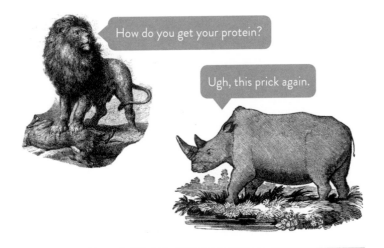

Conversations with non-vegans

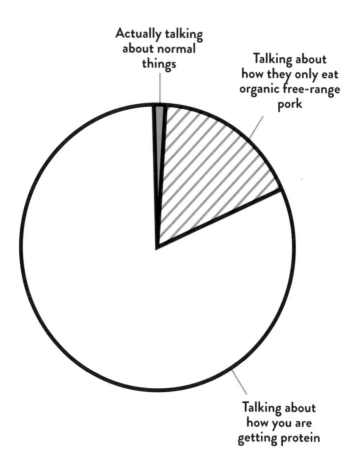

History of vegetarianism

Let's start at the start, vegetarianism is first mentioned in 500 BC by the "Master of Triangles" Pythagoras. He was part of a cult that advocated benevolance to all living creatures, including humans. Vegetarianism was know as a "Pythagorean diet" for years, up until the modern vegetarian movement began in the mid-1800s.

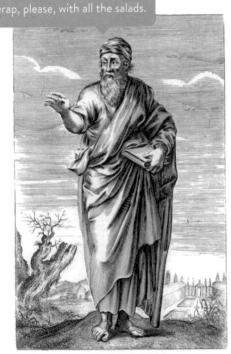

A falafel wrap, please, with all the salads.

PYTHAGORAS.

Humans have, of course, had meatless diets for centuries before Pythagoras. Early humans would have eaten a mainly plant-based diet with a treat of mammoth at Christmas and birthdays.

Many ancient societies had vegetarianism as a commonplace. Buddhism, Hinduism, and Jainism practice vegetarianism, believing that humans should not inflict pain on other animals. India, the home of Hinduism, is still the country with the largest population of vegetarians.

Notable historical vegetarians include:
Leo Tolstoy, George Bernard Shaw, Mahatma Gandhi

Noteable dictators who just happened to be vegetarian:
Adolf Hilter

Are you a dictator?

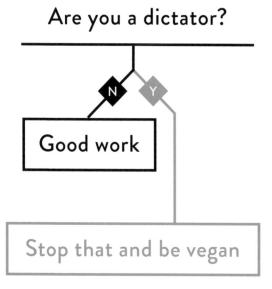

History of veganism

In 1944, Donald Watson, a prominent vegetarian, coined the term "Vegan" as a way to separate vegetarianism with those who also avoided **all** animal products.

Donald's other suggestions included "dairyban," "vitan," and "benevore." Luckily he settled on vegan as vegans get criticized enough without having to be called "dairyban!"

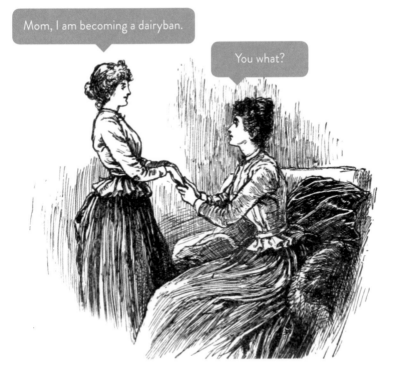

Mom, I am becoming a dairyban.

You what?

The beginning

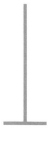

Veg {etari} an

The end

What is a vegan?

Simply put, a vegan is someone who abstains
from eating or using animal products.

Vegans have decided that they can live their lives without
using animal products. There are many reasons to be vegan:
ethics, health, environmental, and bragging rights on Instagram.
Whatever the reason, chosing not to kill animals for your dinner
is a positive choice and one to be applauded.

Being vegan isn't about: gluten free, being healthy,
yoga, clean living, or being nice to people. You can be any of those
things and still be a vegan, but the general public are simply
awful and being nice to them is a chore.

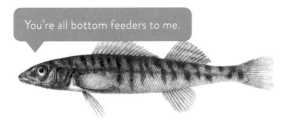

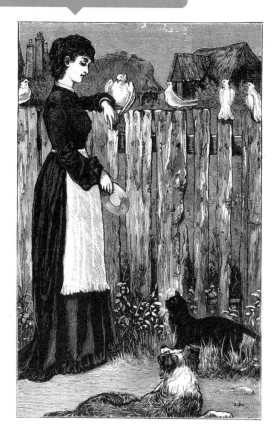

Veganism levels

You can just be a standard vegan, avoiding animal products and living your life. Or you can go extra, outdoing all the other vegans:

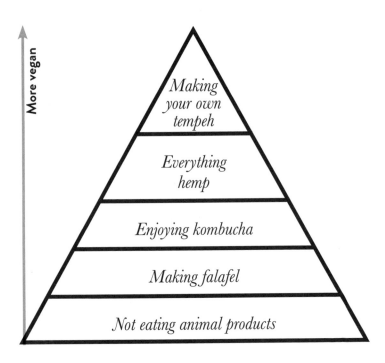

More vegan

Making your own tempeh

Everything hemp

Enjoying kombucha

Making falafel

Not eating animal products

Who eats what?

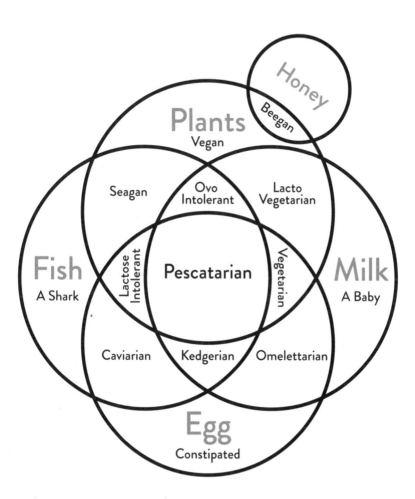

Honey

Plants

Beegan

Vegan

Seagan

Ovo
Intolerant

Lacto
Vegetarian

Fish

Lactose
Intolerant

Pescatarian

Vegetarian

Milk

A Shark

A Baby

Caviarian

Kedgerian

Omelettarian

Egg

Constipated

LET FOOD BE THY MEDICINE

Hypocrates

BUT BACON THO' LOL!

Hilarious internet meat-eater

Do you eat . . .

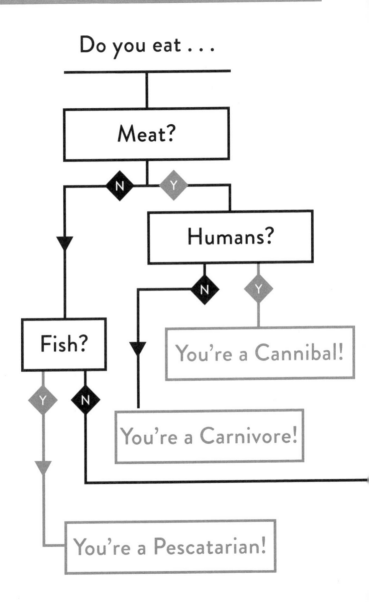

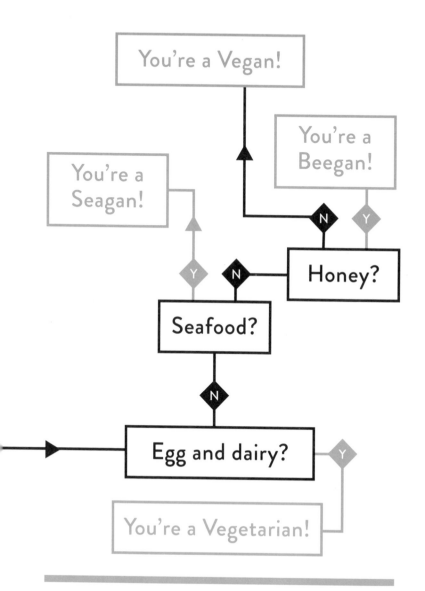

Nomenclature

There are a few synonyms for things in the vegan world. Terms like plant-based and vegan-friendly have started appearing on products. It's a softer way to say "vegan" for those who are a bit squeamish about these things. But being vegan is more than just having a plant-based diet, it's also against the use of animals in all things from clothing to testing cosmetics.

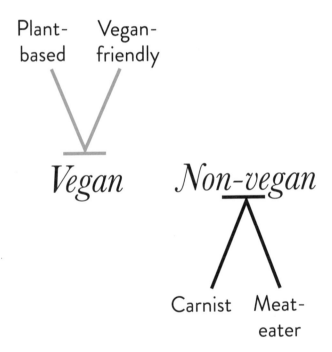

Types of vegan

Because there are many reasons to go vegan there are all sorts of sub-genres of vegan. For example, some vegans are primarily "in it for the animals" without any regard for their own health, while others are concerned more with their carbon footprint.

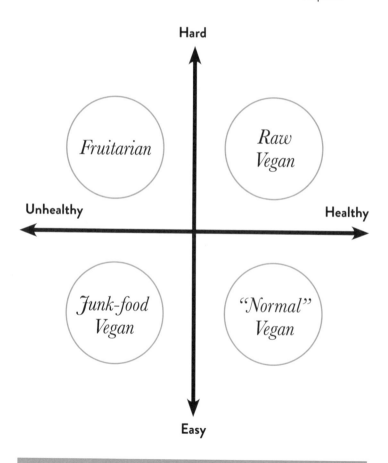

Raw vegans

Rather than this being a cannibalism issue, a raw vegan eats all their food raw or heated to a temperature below 104°–118°F. No processed foods but tons of fruits, vegetables, nuts, seeds, sprouted grains, and legumes.

A raw vegan diet is great for heart health but can cause complications if you don't keep an eye on nutrition. Especially vitamin B12, vitamin D, and calcium.

On the other hand, there are the fruitarians. The fruitarian diet relies on only eating fruit. This will turn your guts into a leaking rusty tap—best to avoid.

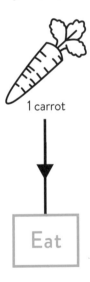

1 carrot

Eat

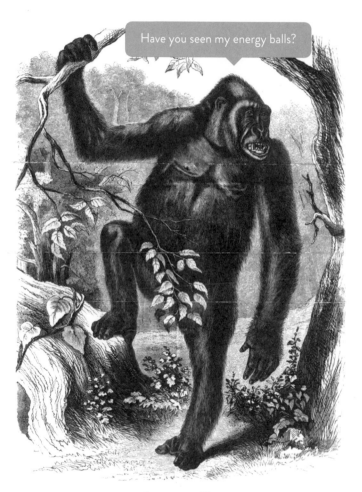

A raw gorilla

Junk-food vegan

Relatively new on the vegan scene, junk-food vegans worship at the temple of seitan and hold all things beige with great regard.

By eating from the beige buffet the junk-food vegans prove that vegan food doesn't have to be healthy or even prolong your life.

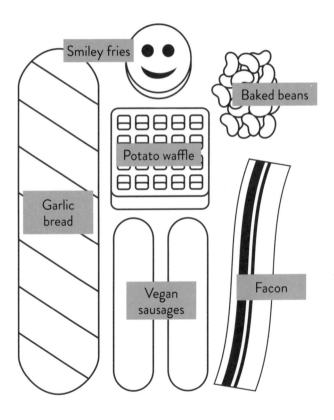

Smiley fries

Baked beans

Potato waffle

Garlic bread

Vegan sausages

Facon

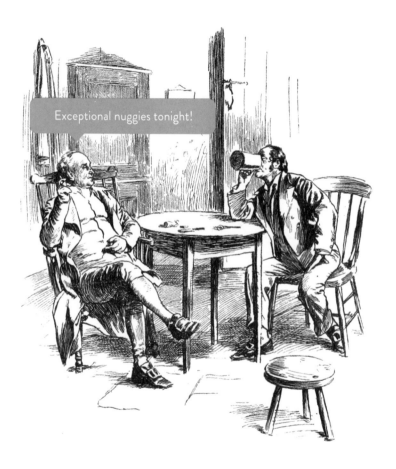

After feasting on breaded items, the junk-food vegans retire to the nuggatorium

The stepping stones to veganism

Jumping head first into veganism can be hard and more than a little daunting. Many people find their route to veganism is:

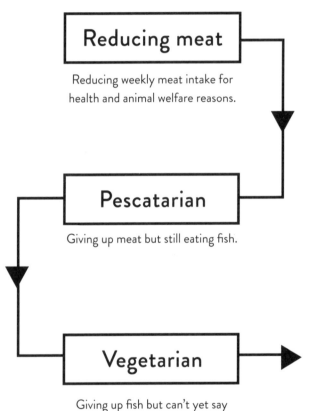

Reducing meat

Reducing weekly meat intake for health and animal welfare reasons.

Pescatarian

Giving up meat but still eating fish.

Vegetarian

Giving up fish but can't yet say goodbye to a cheese omelette.

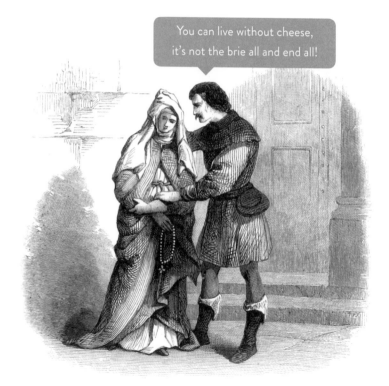

The Instagram effect

The social media platform has been credited with the most
recent rise in veganism, and with the #vegan hashtag on
Instagram having over 85 million results you can see why.
Beautiful images of delicious vegan food are breaking the
perception with painfully cool young people that vegan
food is boring, but more than that it's an aspiration.

Which of us doesn't loving showing off when they've
bothered to arrange vegetables in a bowl?

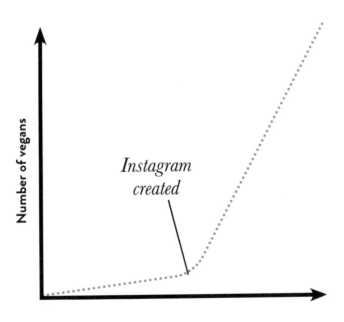

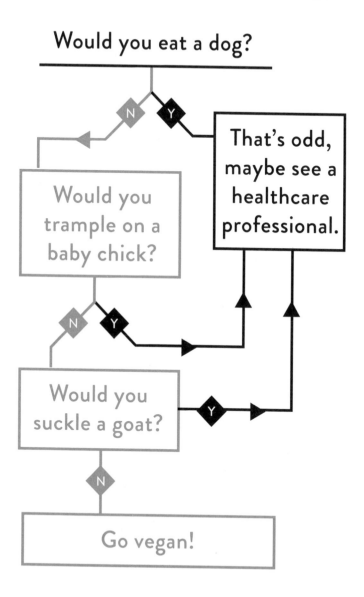

Would you eat a dog?

EACH DAY, A PERSON WHO EATS A VEGAN DIET SAVES:

1
ANIMAL'S
LIFE

44	1,100	22
LBS OF GRAIN	GALLONS OF WATER	LBS OF CO_2

Being vegan

Learn how to live, breathe,
talk, and defecate like a vegan.

Being vegan

Being a vegan isn't all about what you eat. It is mostly about correcting misinformed people in bars that, no, if you don't eat the cows they won't take over the planet, no, you don't need animal protein to live.

Your life choices and dietary decisions are, in their mind, something they feel they have a right to discuss and critique. So equip yourself with the right facts and witty comebacks for when someone inevitably says, "BUT BACON LOL."

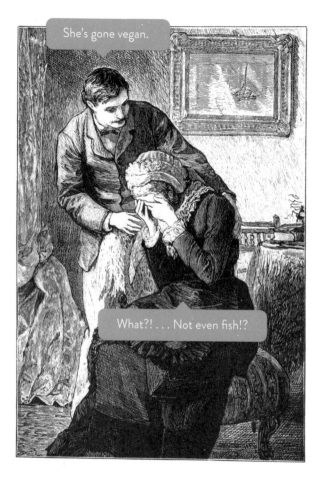

**Sarah's parents as they find out from Instagram
that their beloved daughter has "gone vegan"**

Vegan bingo

Talking about being a vegan with non-vegans?
Expect to hear some of these common phrases:

Can you have gluten?	Do you miss cheese?	You need animal protein to live	We have canines for a reason
Do you want farm animals to go extinct?	Try some, I won't tell anyone	I'm eating double meat to cancel you out	Bacon
I only eat organic meat	Veganism is too extreme	We are top of the food chain	Where do you get your protein?
Lions eat meat	Avocados aren't vegan	Vegetarian is an old name for a bad hunter	What would you do on a desert island?
Figs aren't vegan	Plants have feelings	Cavemen ate meat	Animals are delicious

Winning arguments

The first rule of winning arguments about veganism is that nobody really wins arguments like this, especially online. You're not going to convince a meat eater to go vegan by showing them a nasty video, presenting the facts, or appealing to their compassion for animals. The best strategy is to offer up some simple answers to the more silly questions and then get on with living your vegan-life. Show them by "doing" that living a vegan lifestyle is easy, possible, and you can be mostly normal.

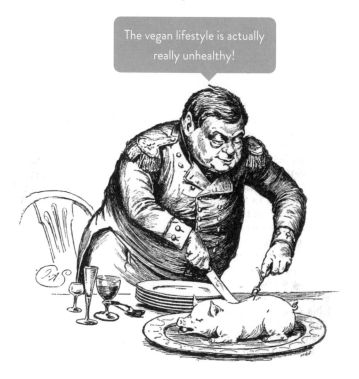

Top "swap" tips for starting out as a vegan

1. Meatless Monday
Make Mondays meat-free

2. Make one meal every day vegan
Start easy, breakfast can be as simple as toast with dairy-free spread or jam.

3. Veganize your usual meals
Swap butter for vegan spread or swap milk for soy.

4. Choose the vegan option on a menu
Chain restaurants are upping their vegan options at the moment: give them a try. If they are awful just order some chips on the side.

5. Replace meat with fake meat/tofu

Stick to your usual "meat and two veg" but swap the meat out for a vegan sausage, or fry up some tofu and cover it in condiments.

6. Add more vegetables

Not only is eating more vegetables better for you (it's the roughage, it aids "digestive transit") but eating half a plate of vegetables with dinner is a great way to reduce meat because there just isn't enough space on the plate for anything else!

7. Follow a vegan

Instagram and Twitter are packed full of pretentious vegan influencers pretending that they are fine functioning members of society. They're not, of course, but they give out great salad tips.

Adjusting your language

After a lifetime of meaty metaphors and animal analogies,
it is time to upgrade your language!

Meat-eaters say	Vegans say
I've got a beef with you	I'm about to go bananas on you
Going cold turkey	Turning over a new leaf
No spring chicken	Salad days are over
Bring home the bacon	The breadwinner
Chicken and egg	Carrot and stick
Like a headless chicken	Full of beans
Chicken feed	Small potatoes

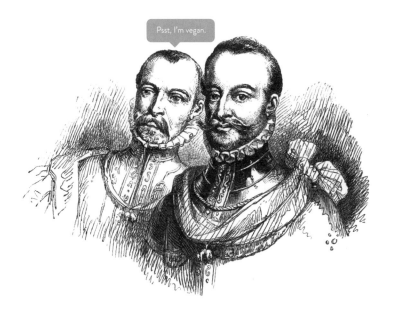

Going to dinner parties

There is no way around it, as a vegan you are now
an awkward dinner-party guest. Congratulations.

You will see your dinner-party invites diminish. But because most
dinner parties are awful, you've done yourself a massive favor.
You no longer have to spend four hours with morons asking you
about protein sources.

If you do get an invite and decide to go, prepare for stuffed peppers,
something with cheese because they forgot that cheese is made
with milk, and a fruit salad for dessert. Best to grab a bag of chips
on the way there to stop your stomach grumbling.

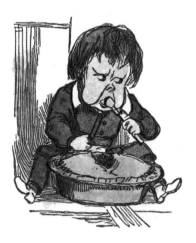

**When you find the one thing
you can eat at the buffet**

Are you a picky eater?

- **N**
- **Y** → **Don't go to the dinner party**

Do you like people?
- **Y**
- **N**

Go to the dinner party

Easy mushroom pâté

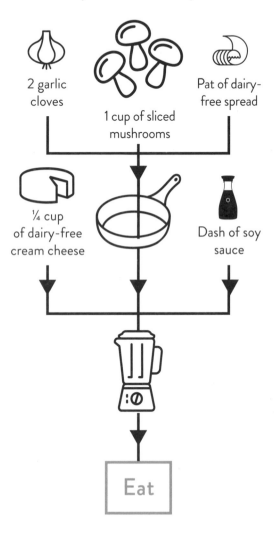

2 garlic
cloves

1 cup of sliced
mushrooms

Pat of dairy-
free spread

¼ cup
of dairy-free
cream cheese

Dash of soy
sauce

Eat

Hosting dinner parties

If you are completely insane you will hold a dinner party and invite non-vegans. It will serve you well to hold off telling people that a dish is vegan until after they have tried it. Nothing will put non-vegans off a dish quicker than knowing it's been made without a hunk of animal.

You can surprise non-vegans by making something unexpectedly vegan, like mac and cheese, and announcing it with a flourish to amaze and astound. But if you're not a great cook and have made a bowl of slop, don't wait too long for your round of applause.

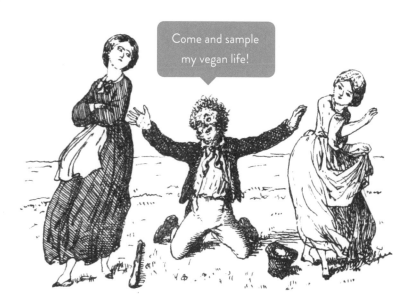

What you wear

It's not just what goes in your mouth that makes you vegan,
it's also the clothes on your back.

There are the more obvious items like leather, suede, wool, and
fur. Silk is often overlooked, as are the feathers in your pillow.
All are obtained through cruelty.

You can easily live without these things; synthetic alternatives are
readily available and just fine.

Maybe don't throw out that leather belt just yet, but look for
alternatives when it's time to replace it. Your crocodile shoes,
on the other hand, need to stay in the past.

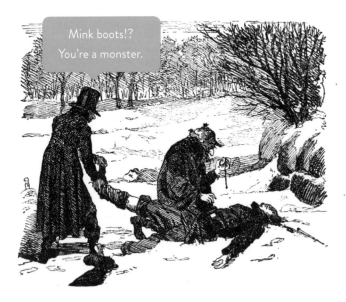

Leather → *PVC leather*

Sorry, you will need to upgrade your jumpsuit.

Fur → *Artificial fur*

Fur? It's not 1970, you don't need fur.

Down → *Artificial down*

Alternatives to feather-filled pillows and
duvets are affordable and easily found.

Eating out

Fully vegan restaurants are few and far between. Even if you do find one, it might be one of the old-school vegan ones where they put seeds and healthy things in everything because that's what they did in the 70s.

If you find yourself in a modern nice restaurant, chances are that there will be a vegan option or at least a meal that is adaptable. Ask for the vegan menu and, if there isn't one, then ask for the allergy menu and you can piece together a meal from there.

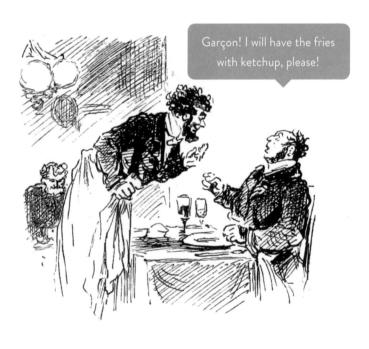

Cuisine	What to eat	Watch out for
Chinese	Sweet and sour tofu, plain rice	Good luck, meat and egg are hidden everywhere . . .
French	er . . . fries?	There is fat in everything, avoid
Indian	Vegetable curry, vegetable samosa, rice, chapatti, or roti	Ask for no ghee, Naan breads contain yogurt
Italian	Pizza with no cheese, pasta and tomato sauce	Fresh pasta will be made with egg
Japanese	Vegetable sushi	Sometimes served with mayo
Middle Eastern	Falafel, hummus, flatbreads	Hidden honey
Thai	Thai curry and coconut rice	Fish sauce can be in the curry paste

This is of course a very rough guide; always ask if a dish is vegan.

WHERE DO I GET MY PROTEIN?

BITCH, PEAS'

Smugness

People find vegans act smug, pretentious, and superior to everyone else. The uncomfortable truth is that vegans are in fact better than everyone else. Vegans have had a look at their lives, made some ethical choices, and they are saving animals and the planet on a daily basis.

People hate vegans because they know they've made decent choices and they just can't bring themselves to do it as well.

So yes, vegans are smug.
It's time to work on your smugface.

Are you better than other people?

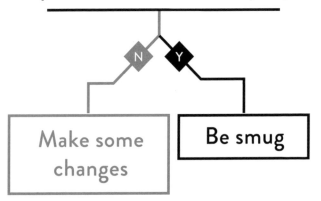

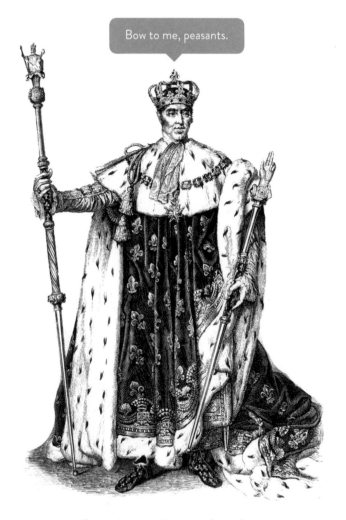

**Stepping out in your faux furs
to defend your way of life**

The "island" and other things that will never happen

You've either already been asked about the "island" or you soon will be. To recap, you will be asked if you are on a desert island with a knife and nothing to eat but a pig, would you kill the pig?

It's basically a spectacular waste of everyone's time. A hypothetical situation that is designed to test your moral boundaries. There are several replies that are useful:

1. What if you're not on the island?
Would you still be wearing a grass skirt, killing pigs with rusty knives in your garden?

2. If you were on the moon with only a pot pie and a spoon, would you eat the pot pie?
No, because that situation is ridiculous.

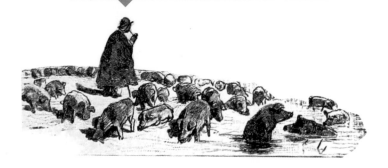

What are the chances that I would land on Pig Island?

You will also find at least one meat-eater claiming they will eat double the amount of meat to cancel you out. Forever. Take a moment to appreciate the time, money, and effort that would take.

Literally eating two steaks every time they want just one. They will be dead within a year.

Amount they were going to eat	**What they have to eat to cancel you out**
	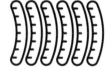
300 calories *$3.00*	*600 calories* *$6.00*
280 calories *$9.00*	*560 calories* *$18.00*

Bowels

As a vegan you're going to naturally be eating a lot more vegetables, and therefore fiber. Animal products don't contain fiber. All that wonderful fiber is going to revolutionize your time in the bathroom.

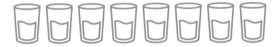

Your body weight (lb) x 0.5 = Water you need every day (oz)

Make sure you're drinking enough water to accompany all this new fiber. To find out how much water to drink, divide your body weight by two, then divide by eight to find the number of glasses you should drink everyday.

Soon enough your "chocolate snakes" will begin to sail through with virtually no resistance. Listen to non-vegans complain about stubborn bowels while you sit back and set your watch to yours. Bliss.

The stinky elephant in the room is flatulance. Vegans fart more than meat-eaters. It's to do with the beans and lentils. Meat-eaters farts do smell much worse though, as the eggs and meat in their guts breaks down to create hydrogen sulphide, or in other words, rotten egg gas!

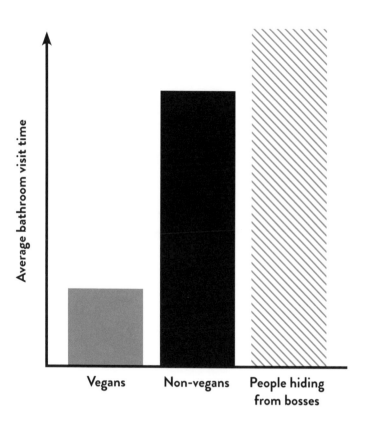

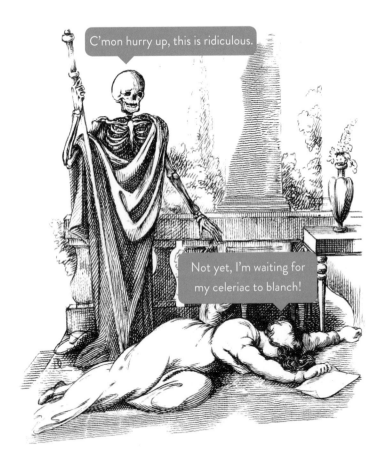

**Death patiently waiting for the
vegans to finish a "Yotam" recipe**

Living longer

Vegans live, on average, six to nine years longer than meat-eaters. With the reduction in consumption of saturated fat and cholesterol, vegans tend to have a reduced risk of heart disease and cancer. The increased life span may be due to the health benefits of a plant-based diet but there is also evidence that vegans are the type of people that make good life choices.If you're reading this with a belly full of doughnuts and the remnants of a hangover, then you're probably the exception to that rule.

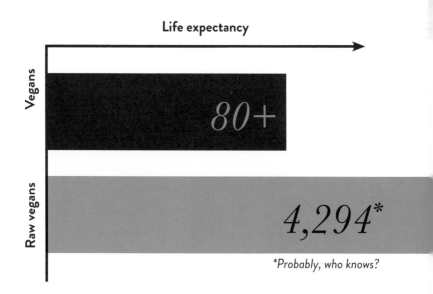

Life expectancy

Vegans
80+

Raw vegans
*4,294**

Probably, who knows?

The vegan police

The vegan police are a tiresome collection of people ready to point out your failings and flaws. You might also experience non-vegans on the other side of the fence pointing out that you used a plastic straw or that you took a flight this year. Well fuck them all.

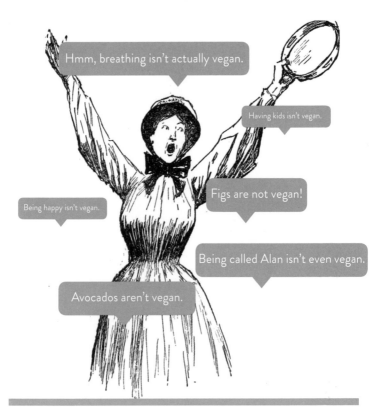

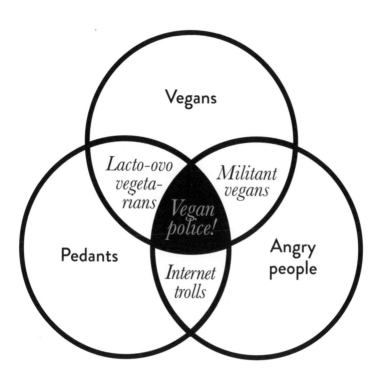

Not being perfect

There is no such thing as a perfect vegan.

However well you are doing at being vegan, there will be something that will trip you up. Maybe something you didn't realize wasn't vegan or maybe you just had to have a bacon sandwich.

The important thing to remember is not to worry, veganism isn't all or nothing. You are doing "something" rather than "nothing." Go you.

You ate something not vegan?

Shake it off and keep on

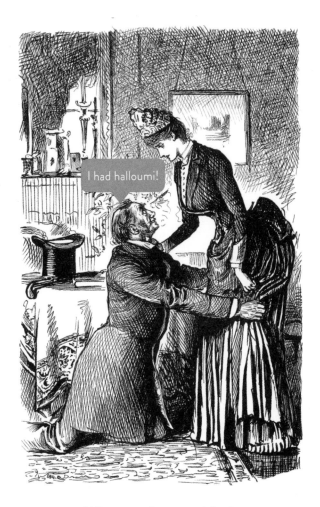

When you have to visit the
vegan queen to ask forgiveness

Shopping vegan

How to spend
your "green" dollars.

Shopping vegan

Myth one, veganism is expensive.

It can be, if you're eating processed foods with every meal. Beans, rice, potatoes, and vegetables are the cheapest things in the supermarket.

Lentils
$0.25

Steak
$8.00

Myth two, veganism is all about being healthy.

It really isn't. You will find unhealthy vegan options everywhere.

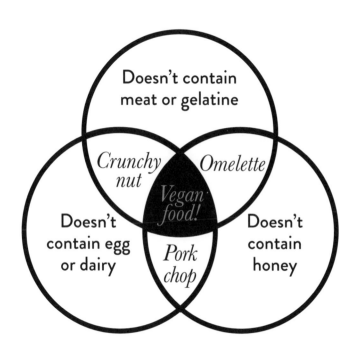

Reading packaging

Obviously the easiest thing to look for is a "Vegan" symbol or for the words "Vegan-friendly." This latter option seems to be a signal to non-vegans that the food in question is not just targeted at healthy vegan hippies, and may still taste good.

Reading packaging at speed is a skill found in vegans and those with allergies. You can find vegans excitedly finding new products in stores and flipping them over to digest the delicious information on the back.

You are looking for three main types of ingredients: hidden meat, hidden dairy (milk and egg), and finally honey.

1. The meat route might be obvious; if you're looking at pork rinds then you're a fool. But also, many meat-flavored chips don't actually contain meat. So the words you are looking for are:
Suitable for vegetarians.

2. Now to hunt out the dairy: allergens like **egg** and **milk** should be in bold in the ingredients.

3. Honey: this one is easier, look for the word **honey.**

4. **May contain traces of . . .**
This means that the ingredient hasn't been deliberately included in the recipe but there may be trace amounts in the product. It doesn't tell you how likely it is to contain the ingredient and it's mainly a warning for allergy sufferers.

Graham Crackers

INGREDIENTS

Flour (56%) (**Wheat**, Calcium, Iron, Niacin, Thiamin), Vegetable Oil, Sugar, Wholemeal **Wheat** Flour (13%), Partially Inverted Sugar Syrup, Gelatin, Raising Agents (Sodium Bicarbonate, Malic Acid, Ammonium Bicarbonate), Salt, Skimmed **Milk** Powder.

Contains: **Milk**

May contain traces of egg and tree nuts

Gelatin? WTF!?

Milk

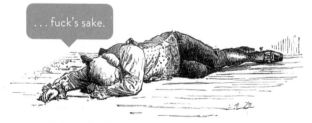

. . . fuck's sake.

Reaching the bottom of the ingredients list and seeing "skimmed milk powder" as the last ingredient

The vegan aisle

There is a new magical aisle appearing in many supermarkets: the vegan aisle. It's a great place to start replacing some non-vegan items like fake meats and to browse for tofu in safety. These aisles can be full of processed foods and can also be expensive, so make sure you visit the vegetable section as well. The lure of some new vegan "steaks" might be great, but remember to stock up on hummus too!

Another great section to visit in the supermarket is the "free-from" section; here you will find many vegan foods, but beware—not all free-from foods are vegan. You won't be the first vegan to excitedly pick up a dairy-free cake to realize it contains egg.

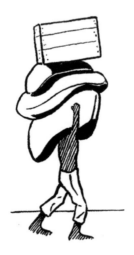

**Leaving the vegan aisle after
a fresh delivery of "facon"**

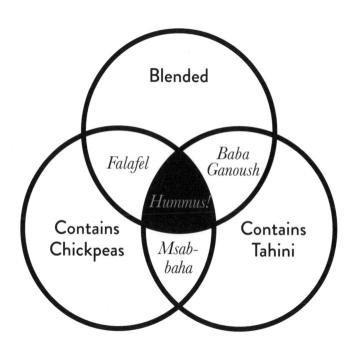

Hidden ingredients

Even the most diligent vegan can miss or overlook non-vegan ingredients. All of these are animal derived: beeswax, down, fur, leather and suede, hide glue, horsehair, lard, rennet, royal jelly, silk, tallow, and wool.

And some of the less obvious ones that sound like they are from the pantry of a Roald Dahl villain: ambergris, bone char, emu oil, and shark fin oil.

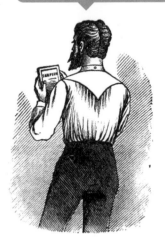

What does it say on the label?	What is it?	Where would I find it hidden?
Carmine (cochineal) or carminic acid	Ground-up insects	Juices, candy, and fizzy drinks
Casein	Milk protein	Processed foods
Gelatin	Cartilage, tendons, fat, and skin of animals	Marshmallows, yogurt, and chewy candy
Isinglass	Air bladders of fish	Wine and beer
Lactose	Milk sugar	Processed foods
Oleic acid	Animal fats	Candy, ice cream, and condiments
Lutein	Yellow coloring from egg yolks	Yellow things
Stearic acid	Animal fats	Baked goods

"Accidentally" vegan snacks

Chips, snacks, and savory items	
SkinnyPop Popcorn*	Vegemite
Lay's (salt & vinegar, bar-b-que, classic, deli style, limon, kettle cooked original, kettle cooked sea salt, cracked black pepper)	Nissin Top Ramen (soy sauce flavor)
Sun Chips (original)	Peanut butter*
Doritos* (spicy sweet chili)	
Ritz crackers	Smiley fries
Triscuits*	Potato waffles
Nabisco Grahams	Potato cakes
Pringles (original, paprika, BBQ and smokey bacon)	Campbell's mushroom gravy
Snyder's jalapeño pretzels	Country Crock plant butter

Some not all, check the packaging to be sure.

The vegan cookie jar

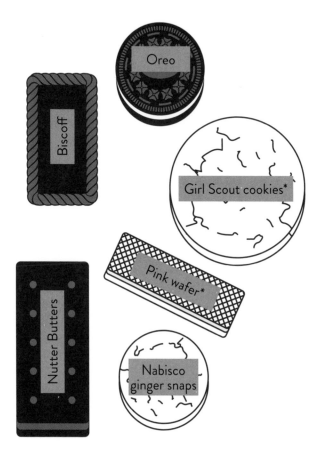

Some not all, check the packaging to be sure

Drinks
LaCroix sparkling water
Ghiradelli hot chocolate mix
Nesquik powder

Candy and pastry	
Skittles*	Pillsbury pastry (crescent rolls, pie crust, biscuits*)
Starburst*	
Swedish Fish	
Sour Patch Kids	Pepperidge Farms puff pastry
Airheads	Duncan Hines frostings and cake mixes
Life Savers hard candy	
SweeTarts	English muffins
Fruit by the Foot	Breakfast muffins*
Bottle Caps	Fig Newtons
Jolly Ranchers	Strudels*

*Some not all, check the packaging to be sure.

Aquafaba meringue recipe

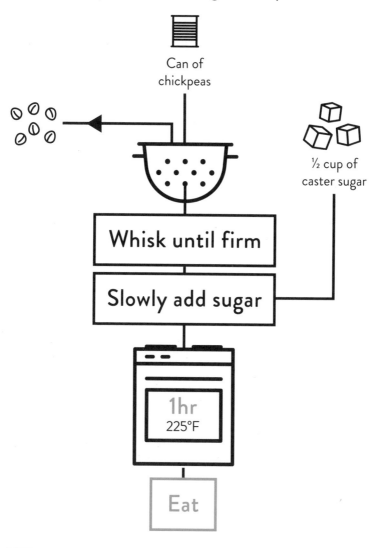

Can of
chickpeas

½ cup of
caster sugar

Whisk until firm

Slowly add sugar

1hr
225°F

Eat

EAT MORE CHIPS

EAT LESS LIPS,

. . EYEHOLES, AND ASSHOLES

The vegan store cupboard

Start filling up your cupboards with easy vegan meals and
ingredients. Dried ingredients like lentils and rice. Introduce
a few at a time rather than changing everything overnight.

What you need	What you need it for
Nutritional yeast or "Nooch"	Making cheese sauces
Liquid smoke	Makes things taste like bacon
Dark chocolate	It's chocolate!
Field Roast sausages	A freezer staple
Waffle fries	Why let kids have all the fun?
Sauerkraut	Fermented cabbage, what's not to like . . .
Sriracha mayo*	Put it on anything
Easy egg replacement	Scrambled "eggs"!

*Not all variants, always check the recipe.

Easy Dhal

Salt

1 cup of
red lentils

2 cups of
water

3 cloves
of garlic

Spices
(1 tsp turmeric
2 tsp cumin seeds
1 tsp garam masala)

Eat

Eating vegan

How to make plants interesting.

Eating vegan

Vegans have come a long way since the 70s stereotypes of mung beans and lentils. Vegans now have chia seeds, mung beans, and lentils, hurrah!

Look forward to hummus being one of your favorite foods, closely followed by baba ganoush and oh, sausage rolls, vegans have got sausage rolls now!

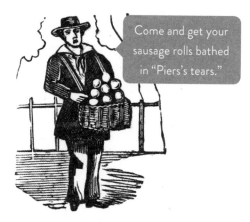

Come and get your sausage rolls bathed in "Piers's tears."

What they think vegans eat

What vegans actually eat

BREAKFAST

Sprouted millet, activated almonds, and a spirulina smoothie

Toast or cereal

LUNCH

A leaf

Baked potato and beans

DINNER

Cultured salad with grains, dust, and sadness

Mac 'n' cheese

Easy Vegemite rolls

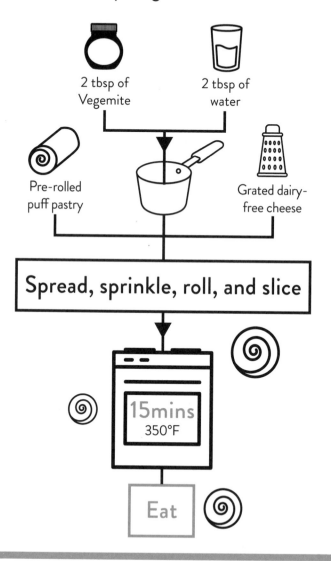

2 tbsp of Vegemite

2 tbsp of water

Pre-rolled puff pastry

Grated dairy-free cheese

Spread, sprinkle, roll, and slice

15mins
350°F

Eat

Vitamin B12

Vitamin B12, also known as cobalamin, is an important vitamin.
It plays an essential role in the production of your red blood cells
and DNA, as well as the functioning of your nervous system.
In short, you need it or you die.

Unfortunately, vitamin B12 is naturally found in meat and dairy.
However, it can also be found in products fortified with B12,
such as some varieties of bread and plant-based milk.

You can't move around a supermarket without falling over
foods fortified with B12. Non-dairy milks and yogurts, cereals,
and nutritional yeast are all dripping with the stuff. You need at
least three micrograms of B12 a day from fortified foods, or if you
wish you can take a weekly B12 supplement providing
at least 2,000 micrograms.

Another great source is a spread that's brown, you either
love it or hate it and it rhymes with carmite. It's Vegemite.
You can buy it at World Market or online.

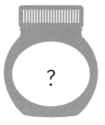

Milk

Vegans don't drink milk that comes from cows, goats, pigs, yaks, or tigers, but that's because no one is brave enough to milk the tigers.

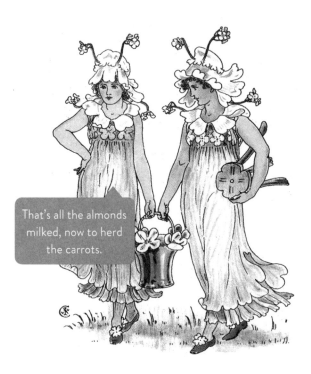

That's all the almonds milked, now to herd the carrots.

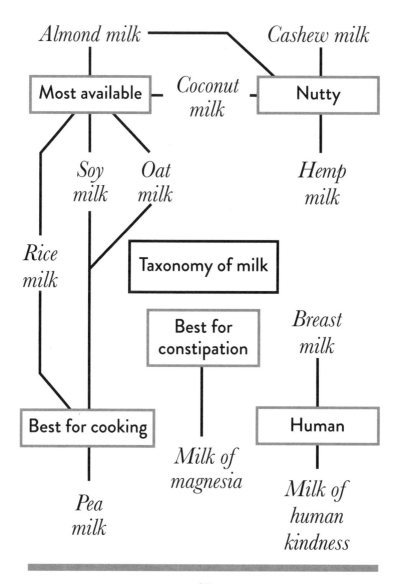

Calcium

We have been conditioned for years that for healthy bones we need to drink cow's milk. Our bones are made from and need the magic ingredient, calcium.

It's easy to overlook that fact that calcium is an element, like hydrogen or mercury. For God's sake don't drink mercury. Calcium is the fifth most abundant element in the Earth's crust and the third most abundant metal. It's literally everywhere. It's not an animal ingredient. **Cows do not make calcium.**

Not only is milk not the best source of calcium, the calcium it does contain isn't as easily absorbed as plant-based calcium. So get your calcium one step further up the chain.

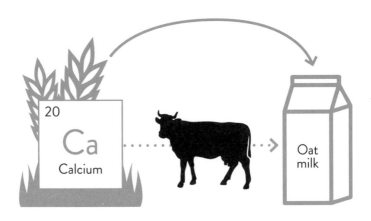

20
Ca
Calcium

Oat milk

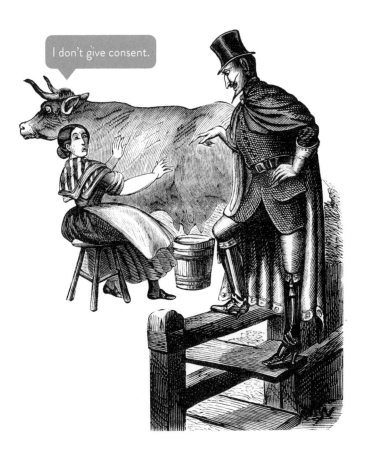

Switching to non-dairy milk

So how do you switch to non-dairy milk? It's really very easy:
buy non-dairy milk, then consume it.

It might take a few days to adjust to the flavor, so try soy or oat
milk first as they are the most bland . . . mmm bland! The nut milks
like almond and coconut are great if you like the flavor of
almond or coconut. Obviously.

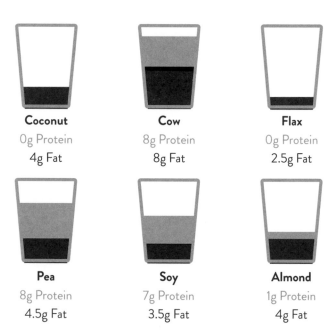

Coconut
0g Protein
4g Fat

Cow
8g Protein
8g Fat

Flax
0g Protein
2.5g Fat

Pea
8g Protein
4.5g Fat

Soy
7g Protein
3.5g Fat

Almond
1g Protein
4g Fat

Crying over split milk?

Make your tea/coffee

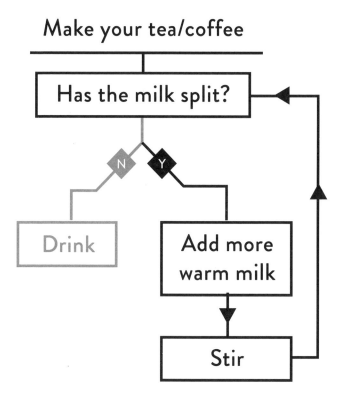

Easy white sauce

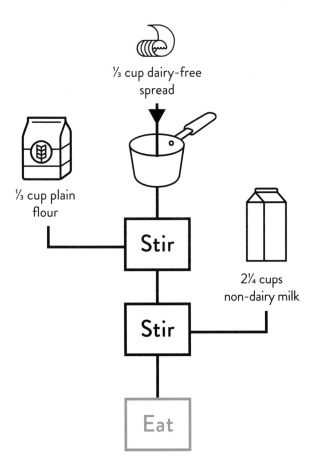

⅓ cup dairy-free spread

⅓ cup plain flour

Stir

2¼ cups non-dairy milk

Stir

Eat

Easy rice pudding recipe

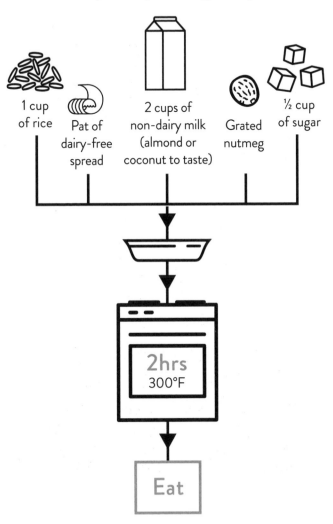

1 cup of rice

Pat of dairy-free spread

2 cups of non-dairy milk (almond or coconut to taste)

Grated nutmeg

½ cup of sugar

2hrs
300°F

Eat

HONEY IS

MADE BY BEES

MAPLE SYRUP IS

MADE BY TREES

Cheese

Cheese, the last refuge of the vegetarian before the vegans drag them into the grand vegan crypt and perform the secret ceremony to rid them of the evilness. There is life after cheese.

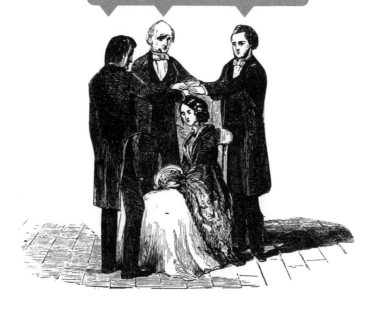

Are you making a cheese sauce?

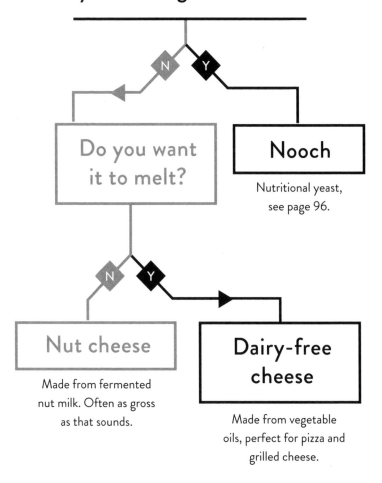

Nooch

Nutritional yeast, see page 96.

Do you want it to melt?

Nut cheese

Made from fermented nut milk. Often as gross as that sounds.

Dairy-free cheese

Made from vegetable oils, perfect for pizza and grilled cheese.

Nooch

Nooch or, to give its full name, nutritional yeast is made from deactivated yeast that fermented on top of a puddle of molasses, ooh yummy!

If you can ignore the weird name and the fact it looks like fish food, nooch is actually delicious and full of wonderful dusty goodness, namely vitamin B12. It's nutty, cheesy flavor is perfect for cheese sauces or just sprinkling on dull vegetables. It will soon be a vegan staple that you can't live without.

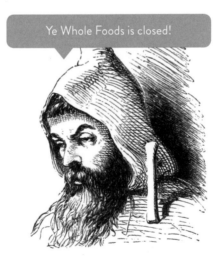

Ye Whole Foods is closed!

When you've run out of nooch and it's medieval England and nooch hasn't been invented yet

Easy vegan mac and cheese

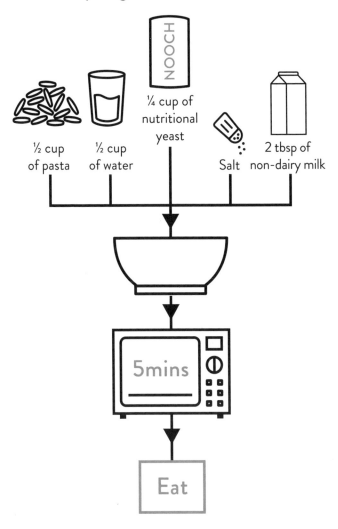

¼ cup of nutritional yeast

½ cup of pasta

½ cup of water

Salt

2 tbsp of non-dairy milk

5mins

Eat

Eggs

Eggs are easy to replace in baking and can be replaced with varying success in things like omelettes and scrambled eggs. Eating your tofu scramble safe in the knowledge that you're not consigning baby chicks to the mincer? Delicious.

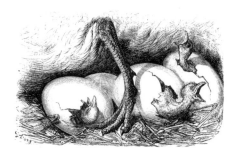

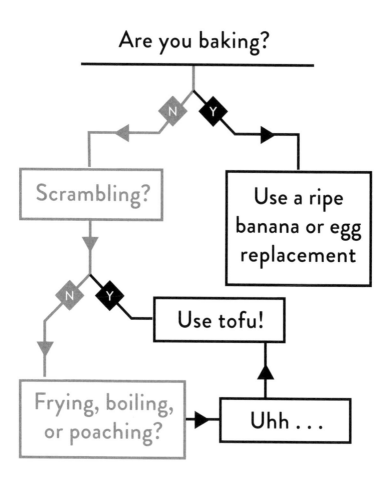

Are you baking?

N   Y

Scrambling?

Use a ripe banana or egg replacement

N   Y

Use tofu!

Frying, boiling, or poaching?

Uhh . . .

Egg recipes

Custard → *Bird's*

By "Bird's" we don't mean birds, we mean Bird's as made
by Mr. Bird. He invented Bird's custard powder because
his wife had an egg allergy, but loved custard.
It's available at World Market or online.

Egg whites → *Aquafaba*

The highest level vegan ingredient, the water from
a can of chickpeas can make meringue. Witchcraft.

Scrambled eggs → *Tofu*

Mash up and fry in a pan. Delicious.

Easy custard tarts

Pepperidge Farms puff pastry cut into circles

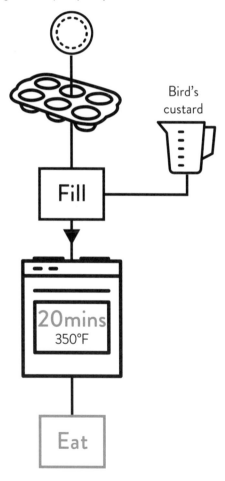

Bird's
custard

Fill

20mins
350°F

Eat

Baking

Vegan baking can be hard. There are various replacements for the critical ingredient, eggs, and some trial and error is required to veganize your favorite baked goods. If you're looking to replace an egg-wash on a pie then simply use oat or soy milk.

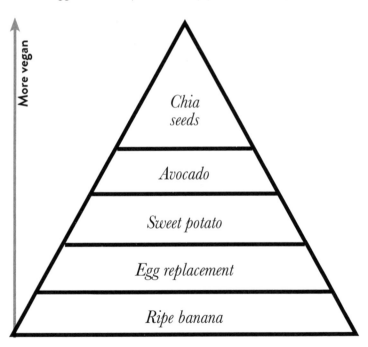

More vegan

Chia seeds

Avocado

Sweet potato

Egg replacement

Ripe banana

Easy pancakes

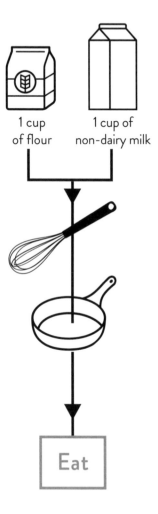

1 cup
of flour

1 cup of
non-dairy milk

Eat

Easy brownie recipe

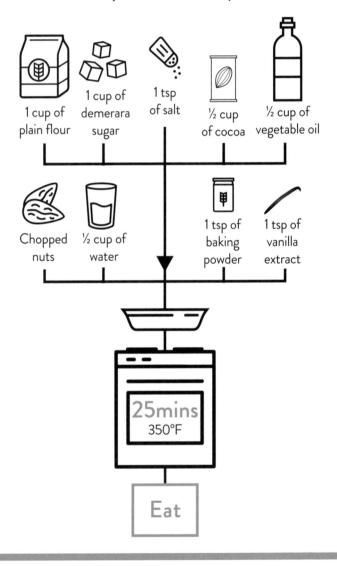

1 cup of plain flour

1 cup of demerara sugar

1 tsp of salt

½ cup of cocoa

½ cup of vegetable oil

Chopped nuts

½ cup of water

1 tsp of baking powder

1 tsp of vanilla extract

25mins
350°F

Eat

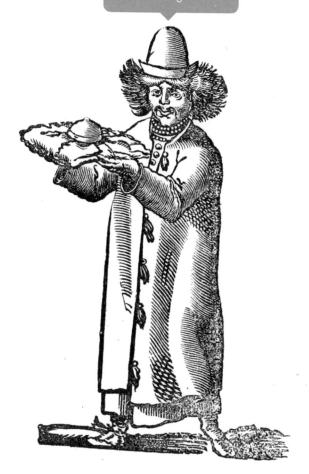

When you make a vegan cake and it
rises and doesn't taste like rubber

Banana bread recipe

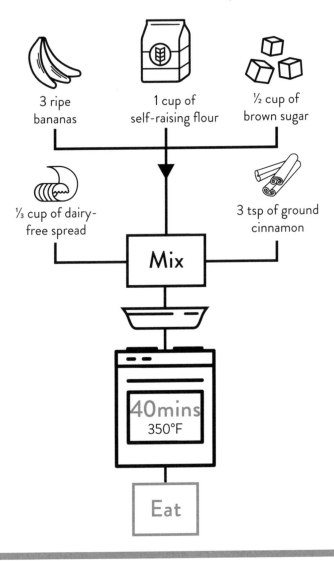

3 ripe
bananas

1 cup of
self-raising flour

½ cup of
brown sugar

⅓ cup of dairy-
free spread

3 tsp of ground
cinnamon

Mix

40mins
350°F

Eat

Cinnamon roll recipe

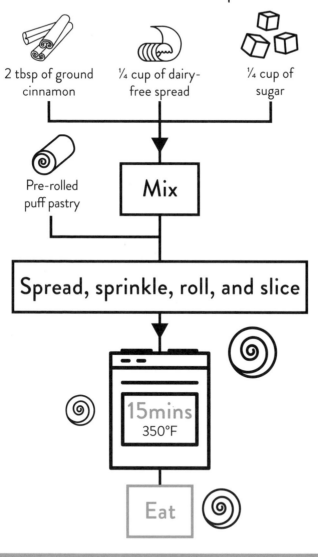

2 tbsp of ground cinnamon

¼ cup of dairy-free spread

¼ cup of sugar

Pre-rolled puff pastry

Mix

Spread, sprinkle, roll, and slice

15mins
350°F

Eat

Anatomy of a potato

The humble potato, is there nothing it can't do?
Potatoes are an excellent source of vitamin C,
have more potassium than a banana, and are a great
source of vitamin B6. Potatoes are also fat and
cholesterol-free (until you deep fry them).

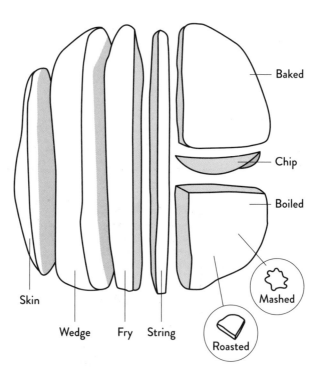

Baked

Chip

Boiled

Skin

Wedge   Fry   String

Roasted

Mashed

Anatomy of a cauliflower

If you're looking for the low-carb version of a potato, look no further than the cauliflower. You can mash cauliflower, slice them into a steak, or blend them into small pieces like rice. However, if you replace everything with cauliflower you will also replace fun with sadness.

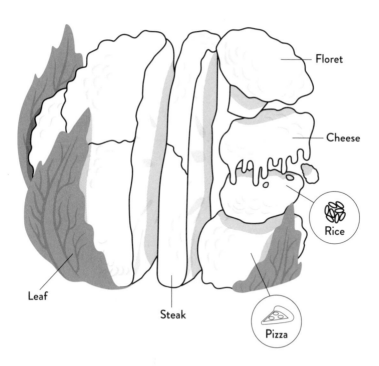

Floret

Cheese

Rice

Leaf

Steak

Pizza

Meat

Vegan sausage rolls are fantastic, but there is nothing more delicious than the tears of a meat-eater when you tell them that a sausage is just a shape and doesn't have to contain meat.

Actually, sausage is derived from the Latin "*salsicus*" meaning "seasoned with salt." Please be my friend.

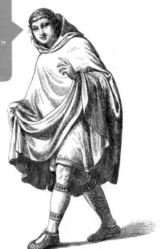

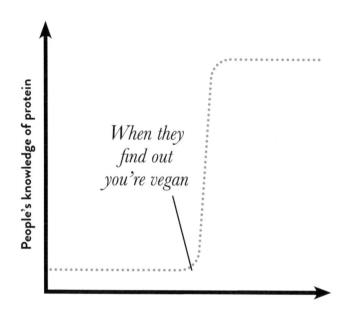

"Fake" meat

There are many types of fake meat made from soy, peas, beans, mycoprotein (a type of fungus), and seitan (wheat gluten). It's like eating science, so exciting!

You'll find non-vegans can be squeamish about some of these products, the irony being that they are happy to eat a hotdog . . .

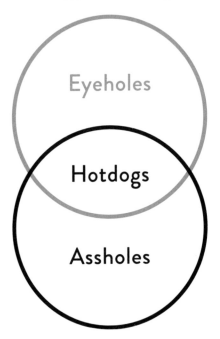

Although much lower in saturated fat, fake meats are processed
foods so eat them as you would any treat, in moderation.

To cook, you can treat these fake meats just like the real thing,
cook on a BBQ, fry in a frying pan, or roast in the oven.
Unlike real meat, you can't undercook them and give
yourself awful food poisoning.

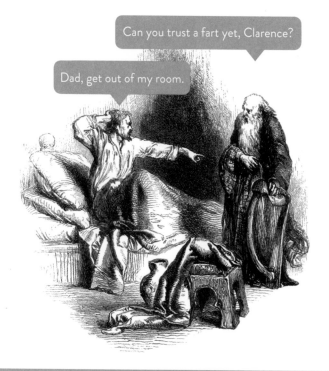

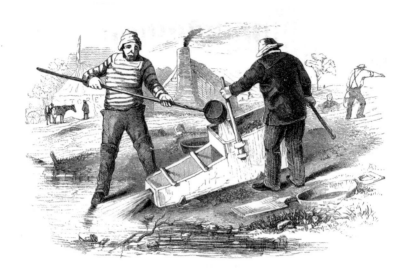

**Month-old tempeh slurry being tipped
into troughs behind The Happy Carrot café,
San Francisco, 1972**

Natural protein sources

Contrary to popular belief, you don't actually need that much protein to live. Even if you are crushing it at the gym, you're not going to struggle on a vegan diet. The word for a protein deficiency is kwashiorkor; you've not heard of it because it's incredibly rare.

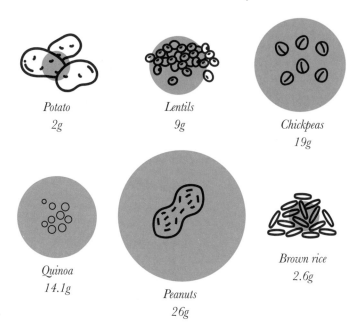

Potato
2g

Lentils
9g

Chickpeas
19g

Quinoa
14.1g

Peanuts
26g

Brown rice
2.6g

Easy tofu stir fry

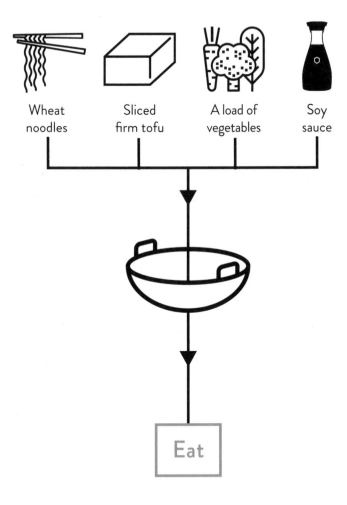

| Wheat noodles | Sliced firm tofu | A load of vegetables | Soy sauce |

Eat

Tofu and tempeh

There are a few types of tofu available: firm, extra firm, silken, and tempeh. The difference between them is how much water they contain. Tofu is pretty tasteless but it acts as a superb sponge for the flavors and sauces you add to it.

Silken tofu
Very soft. Works well in sauces and dressings. Great as a replacement for eggs in baking.

Firm tofu
Firm. Obviously. Works well fried but can be crumbled to make scrambled tofu.

Extra firm tofu
A great replacement for meat. Can be oven baked and fried.

Tempeh
Whole fermented soy beans in a firm cake. Use as you would extra firm tofu.

Roast dinner

The classic roast dinner is actually mostly vegan. Obviously the large chunk of meat is out, but the trimmings are the best bits anyway!

Main event	Sauces
Roast potatoes	Mint sauce
Boiled greens (broccoli, Brussels sprouts)	Mustard
Stuffing	Cranberry sauce
Nut roast or other meat replacement	Vegetable gravy
Roast parsnips	Horseradish
Mashed rutabaga	*Vegan bread sauce
Roast carrots	Applesauce

To make a vegan bread sauce, follow the easy white sauce recipe on page 90 and replace the flour with breadcrumbs.

Easy popovers

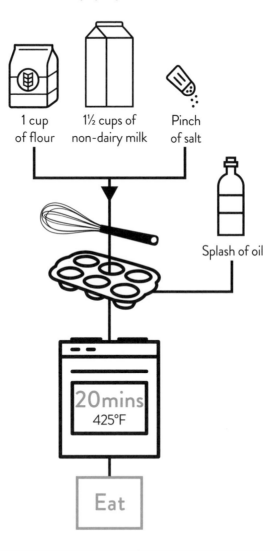

1 cup
of flour

1½ cups of
non-dairy milk

Pinch
of salt

Splash of oil

20mins
425°F

Eat

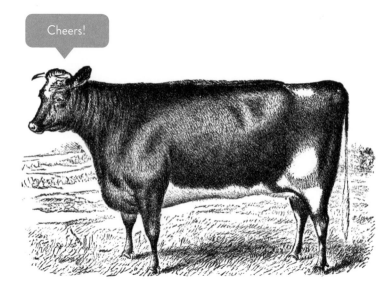

About the author

Stephen Wildish is the author of *How to Swear* and *How to Adult*. He's also a vegan who's teetotal and into CrossFit. He doesn't know what to tell you about first!

Stephen is the current 100m and 200m sack-race world record holder.

He couldn't have written all this nonsense without the help of Jake Allnutt, Jake Yapp, Robert Arnold, Ugly Vegan, Lucie Johnson, Susan Wildish, Ted Wildish, and Lily Wildish.